Weight Bearing Exercises for Osteoporosis

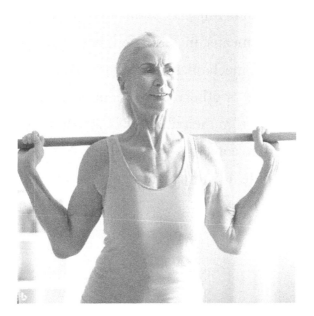

Scientifically Proven Home Exercises to Strengthen Your Bones and Reduce the Risk of Fracture

Patrick Moore

Table of Contents

Introduction

Welcome to "Weight-Bearing Exercises for Osteoporosis: Scientifically Proven Home Exercises to Strengthen Your Bones and Reduce the Risk of Fracture." This book is a comprehensive guide that empowers you to take control of your bone health and combat the challenges posed by osteoporosis through effective weight-bearing exercises.

Osteoporosis is a condition that weakens bones, making them fragile and prone to fractures. It affects millions of people worldwide, predominantly older adults, and can significantly impact their quality of life. However, there is hope. Scientific research has demonstrated the immense benefits of weight-bearing exercises in strengthening bones and reducing the risk of fractures.

In this book, we have compiled a wealth of knowledge and practical exercises to guide you in incorporating weight-bearing exercises into your daily routine. These exercises, backed by scientific evidence, work by stimulating bone cells to rebuild and strengthen your skeletal system. Additionally, they improve muscle strength, balance, and coordination, which are crucial for overall physical well-being.

Throughout the pages of this book, you will explore a variety of low-impact and high-impact weight-bearing exercises tailored to different fitness levels and preferences. From walking, dancing, water aerobics, tai chi, and yoga to jogging, jumping rope, tennis, basketball, and hiking, you will find a range of exercises to suit your individual needs and goals.

Strength-training exercises play a vital role in promoting bone health. You will discover exercises such as bicep curls, squats, lunges, push-ups, and pull-ups that specifically target muscle groups and enhance bone density. Additionally, balance exercises like standing on one leg, practising tai chi and yoga, and walking on a balance beam will improve stability and reduce the risk of falls.

We will guide you in creating a personalised exercise plan, staying motivated, and monitoring your progress along the way. However, it is crucial to consult with your healthcare provider before starting any exercise program, especially if you have pre-existing health conditions or concerns.

Chapter 1

Understanding Osteoporosis

What is Osteoporosis?

Osteoporosis is a progressive skeletal disorder characterised by low bone mass and a deterioration of bone tissue. It is often referred to as the "silent disease" because it develops gradually without causing noticeable symptoms until a fracture occurs. In fact, many individuals may remain unaware of their condition until they experience a bone fracture, which can be a life-altering event.

Within our bodies, bones undergo a continuous process of remodelling. Specialised cells called osteoclasts break down old bone tissue, while osteoblasts generate new bone tissue to replace it. In osteoporosis, the balance between bone breakdown and formation is disrupted, leading to a net loss of bone density and strength over time.

As a result, bones become weak, brittle, and more susceptible to fractures. Even minor stresses or falls that would not normally cause significant harm can result in fractures in individuals with osteoporosis. Common fracture sites include the hips, spine, wrists, and ribs.

Osteoporosis predominantly affects postmenopausal women due to the hormonal changes associated with menopause. However, it can also occur in men and individuals of any age due to various factors, such as certain medications, hormonal imbalances, sedentary lifestyle, inadequate nutrition, and a family history of the disease.

Understanding the risk factors and causes of osteoporosis is crucial for prevention, early detection, and effective management. Regular bone density screenings, lifestyle modifications, and appropriate medical interventions can help reduce the impact of osteoporosis and lower the risk of fractures.

The Impact of Osteoporosis on Bone Health

Osteoporosis has a significant impact on bone health, leading to a gradual deterioration of bone tissue and decreased bone density. Understanding how this condition affects bone health is crucial for grasping the importance of preventive measures and targeted interventions. Here are some key aspects of the impact of osteoporosis on bone health:

1. Decreased Bone Density: Osteoporosis causes a reduction in bone mineral density (BMD), which refers to the amount of minerals, primarily calcium, present in the bones. As bone density decreases, bones become more porous and fragile, increasing the risk of fractures.

2. Weakening of Bone Structure: Osteoporosis affects the microarchitecture of bone, disrupting the intricate network of trabeculae and thinning the cortical bone. These structural changes compromise the strength and integrity of bones, making them susceptible to fractures even from minor trauma or falls.

3. Increased Bone Resorption: Osteoclasts, cells responsible for breaking down old bone tissue, become overactive in individuals with osteoporosis. This excessive bone resorption outpaces the formation of new bone by osteoblasts, resulting in a net loss of bone mass.

4. *Altered Bone Remodelling Process:* In healthy bones, a dynamic balance exists between bone resorption and bone formation, known as the bone remodeling process. Osteoporosis disrupts this equilibrium, leading to an imbalance favouring bone resorption. As a result, bone turnover becomes dysregulated, further contributing to bone loss and decreased bone quality.

5. *Increased Susceptibility to Fractures:* The weakened bones in individuals with osteoporosis are highly susceptible to fractures. Fractures commonly occur in weight-bearing bones such as the hips, spine, and wrists, but they can also affect other bones in the body. Fractures associated with osteoporosis can cause significant pain, disability, and a decline in overall physical function.

The Role of Exercise in Osteoporosis Management

Exercise plays a vital role in the management of osteoporosis by improving bone density, strength, and overall physical function. Incorporating regular exercise into your routine can help mitigate the effects of osteoporosis and reduce the risk of fractures. Here are some key aspects of the role of exercise in osteoporosis management:

1. Stimulating Bone Formation: Weight-bearing exercises, such as walking, dancing, and weightlifting, subject the bones to mechanical stress, which stimulates the osteoblasts to build new bone tissue. This process, known as bone remodeling, helps increase bone density and strength.

2. Improving Muscle Strength: Exercise not only benefits bones but also enhances muscle strength. Strong muscles provide support to the skeletal system and help reduce the risk of falls and fractures. Strength-training exercises, such as resistance training and weightlifting, target specific muscle groups and promote muscle growth, enhancing overall physical strength and stability.

3. *Enhancing Balance and Coordination:* Osteoporosis increases the risk of falls, which can have severe consequences for individuals with weakened bones. Exercise, particularly balance and coordination exercises like tai chi and yoga, can improve postural stability, proprioception, and coordination, reducing the risk of falls and related fractures.

4. *Maintaining Joint Mobility and Flexibility:* Osteoporosis can lead to stiffness and reduced mobility in joints. Regular exercise that incorporates stretching and range-of-motion exercises helps maintain joint flexibility, improve functional movement, and prevent joint limitations.

5. *Boosting Overall Health and Well-being:* Exercise has numerous additional health benefits beyond bone health. It improves cardiovascular fitness, promotes weight management, reduces the risk of chronic conditions such as heart disease and diabetes, and enhances mental well-being. Engaging in regular exercise can improve overall health and quality of life for individuals with osteoporosis.

It is important to note that not all exercises are suitable for individuals with osteoporosis. Certain high-impact activities or movements that involve excessive spinal flexion or twisting may increase the risk of fractures.

Chapter 2

Importance of Weight-Bearing Exercises

Benefits of Weight-Bearing Exercises

Weight-bearing exercises are essential for maintaining bone health and reducing the risk of fractures. These exercises involve activities that require your body to work against gravity while supporting your own weight. Engaging in weight-bearing exercises on a regular basis offers a multitude of benefits that go beyond just strengthening bones. In this chapter, we will explore the importance of weight-bearing exercises and delve into the specific benefits they provide. Let's explore some of these benefits:

1. Increased Bone Density: Weight-bearing exercises stimulate bone formation and help increase bone density. As you subject your bones to impact and resistance, the mechanical stress triggers the production of new bone tissue. Over time, this can lead to stronger, denser bones, reducing the risk of fractures.

2. *Enhanced* *Muscle* *Strength:* Weight-bearing exercises not only benefit your bones but also strengthen the surrounding muscles. These exercises require your muscles to work against gravity, improving muscle strength and power. Strong muscles provide support to the skeletal system, reduce the risk of falls, and improve overall physical function.

3. *Improved* *Balance* *and* *Stability:* Weight-bearing exercises that focus on balance, such as yoga or Tai Chi, improve proprioception and postural stability. By enhancing your balance and stability, you reduce the likelihood of falls and related fractures, especially in individuals with osteoporosis.

4. *Better* *Joint* *Health:* Engaging in weight-bearing exercises helps maintain joint health and mobility. Regular movement and impact stimulate the production of synovial fluid, which lubricates the joints and nourishes the surrounding cartilage. This can help alleviate joint stiffness, reduce the risk of degenerative conditions like osteoarthritis, and improve overall joint function.

5. *Enhanced Coordination and Body Awareness:* Weight-bearing exercises that involve complex movements, such as dance or certain sports, improve coordination and body awareness. These activities require you to coordinate multiple muscle groups and movements, promoting better motor control and overall physical coordination.

6. *Improved Overall Fitness:* Weight-bearing exercises contribute to overall fitness by increasing cardiovascular endurance, promoting weight management, and boosting energy levels. Regular exercise can help reduce the risk of chronic diseases such as heart disease, diabetes, and obesity, while improving overall mental well-being.

How Weight-Bearing Exercises Improve Bone Density

Weight-bearing exercises play a crucial role in improving bone density, which is essential for maintaining strong and healthy bones. When you engage in weight-bearing exercises, you subject your bones to gravitational forces and mechanical stress, stimulating them to become denser and stronger. Here are some key mechanisms through which weight-bearing exercises improve bone density:

1. Bone Remodeling: Weight-bearing exercises trigger a process called bone remodeling. During this process, specialised cells known as osteoblasts and osteoclasts work together to remove old or damaged bone tissue and replace it with new, healthy bone tissue. The mechanical stress placed on the bones during weight-bearing exercises stimulates the osteoblasts to lay down new bone matrix, leading to increased bone density.

2. Increased Bone Formation: Weight-bearing exercises, such as walking, running, or resistance training, create an environment that encourages bone formation. The impact and stress placed on the bones during these exercises signal the osteoblasts to produce more bone tissue. Over time, this increased bone formation helps improve bone density, making the bones stronger and less prone to fractures.

3. ***Improved Calcium Absorption:*** Weight-bearing exercises also enhance the body's ability to absorb and utilise calcium, a vital mineral for bone health. Calcium is a key component of bone tissue, and its adequate intake and absorption are essential for maintaining bone density. Weight-bearing exercises stimulate the bones to become more receptive to calcium, promoting its absorption and incorporation into the bone matrix.

4. ***Increased Muscle Strength:*** Weight-bearing exercises not only benefit bones but also strengthen the muscles that surround and support them. When you engage in activities like weightlifting or resistance training, the muscles pull on the bones, creating tension and stress. This muscle activity stimulates the bones to adapt and become stronger, as they need to withstand the forces exerted by the contracting muscles.

Other Health Benefits of Weight-Bearing Exercises

Engaging in weight-bearing exercises offers a multitude of health benefits beyond improving bone density. These exercises contribute to overall physical well-being and can positively impact various aspects of your health. Let's explore some of the additional health benefits associated with weight-bearing exercises:

1. Cardiovascular Fitness: Weight-bearing exercises that elevate your heart rate, such as jogging, dancing, or playing sports, improve cardiovascular fitness. Regular aerobic activity strengthens your heart, increases lung capacity, and improves the efficiency of oxygen delivery to your muscles and organs. This can help lower the risk of heart disease, improve circulation, and enhance overall cardiovascular health.

2. Weight Management: Weight-bearing exercises can aid in weight management and the prevention of obesity. These exercises burn calories and help build lean muscle mass, which increases your metabolic rate. Regular physical activity combined with a balanced diet can assist in maintaining a healthy weight, reducing the risk of obesity-related conditions such as diabetes, high blood pressure, and certain cancers.

3. Mental Well-being: Weight-bearing exercises have been shown to have a positive impact on mental health. Physical activity releases endorphins, the "feel-good" hormones, which can enhance mood, reduce stress, and alleviate symptoms of anxiety and depression. Engaging in weight-bearing exercises provides an opportunity for relaxation, focus, and the promotion of overall mental well-being.

4. Improved Joint Stability and Flexibility: Weight-bearing exercises that involve movements like squats, lunges, or yoga poses promote joint stability and flexibility. Strengthening the muscles around the joints provides support and helps maintain joint alignment, reducing the risk of injuries and enhancing overall joint function. Additionally, these exercises improve flexibility, allowing for a greater range of motion, which is essential for daily activities and maintaining an active lifestyle.

5. Enhanced Posture and Body Alignment: Weight-bearing exercises contribute to improved posture and body alignment. Strengthening the muscles in your back, abdomen, and lower body helps maintain proper spinal alignment, reducing the risk of postural imbalances and associated discomfort. Good posture not only enhances your physical appearance but also helps prevent back pain and other musculoskeletal issues.

6. *Increased Energy and Stamina:* Regular participation in weight-bearing exercises can increase your energy levels and overall stamina. As you engage in these activities, your body becomes more efficient at utilizing oxygen and nutrients, leading to improved energy production and endurance. With increased stamina, you can perform daily tasks with greater ease and engage in physical activities for more extended periods without fatigue.

Chapter 3

Getting Started with Weight-Bearing Exercises

Consulting with Your Healthcare Provider

Before embarking on any new exercise program, it is essential to consult with your healthcare provider, particularly if you have any underlying health conditions or concerns. Your healthcare provider can offer valuable guidance and ensure that you approach weight-bearing exercises in a safe and appropriate manner. Here are the reasons why consulting with your healthcare provider is important:

1. Assessing Your Current Health Status: Your healthcare provider will evaluate your overall health, taking into consideration factors such as your medical history, existing conditions, medications, and any previous injuries or surgeries. This assessment will help determine if there are any specific exercise precautions or modifications you need to be aware of.

2. Evaluating Bone Health: If you have been diagnosed with osteoporosis or have concerns about your bone health, your healthcare provider can conduct tests to assess your bone density and provide recommendations based on the results. They can also offer insights into any specific considerations for weight-bearing exercises based on your bone health status.

3. Addressing Individual Needs and Limitations: Each person's fitness level and physical capabilities are unique. Your healthcare provider can take into account your individual needs and limitations to provide tailored recommendations for weight-bearing exercises that are safe and suitable for you. They can suggest modifications or alternative exercises to accommodate any physical limitations you may have.

4. Managing Existing Conditions: If you have other health conditions such as arthritis, cardiovascular disease, or joint problems, your healthcare provider can offer advice on how to adapt weight-bearing exercises to accommodate these conditions. They may recommend specific exercises that are less likely to aggravate your condition or provide guidance on appropriate intensity levels.

5. Medication Considerations: Some medications can affect bone health or increase the risk of fractures. Your healthcare provider can review your medication regimen and advise if any adjustments or precautions are necessary when engaging in weight-bearing exercises. They can also provide insights into how exercise may interact with your medications.

6. *Providing Personalised Recommendations:* Based on your health assessment, your healthcare provider can provide personalised recommendations for the type, frequency, and intensity of weight-bearing exercises that are appropriate for you. They can help you set realistic goals and develop an exercise plan that aligns with your capabilities and health objectives.

Assessing Your Fitness Level

Assessing your fitness level is an important step in getting started with weight-bearing exercises. It helps you understand your current physical capabilities, identify areas for improvement, and determine the appropriate starting point for your exercise routine. Here are some key aspects to consider when assessing your fitness level:

1. Aerobic Fitness: Assessing your aerobic fitness level involves evaluating your cardiovascular endurance. This can be done through various methods, such as performing a timed walk or jog, measuring your heart rate recovery after exercise, or using fitness assessment tools like a step test or a treadmill test. The results of these assessments provide insights into your current cardiovascular fitness and help determine the appropriate intensity and duration for your aerobic exercises.

2. Muscular Strength: Evaluating your muscular strength involves assessing the ability of your muscles to exert force against resistance. This can be done through exercises like push-ups, squats, or using weight machines. Assessing your muscular strength helps identify areas of strength and weakness, enabling you to focus on specific muscle groups during your strength-training exercises.

3. Flexibility: Assessing your flexibility involves evaluating the range of motion of your joints and muscles. This can be done through exercises that target different muscle groups, such as stretching exercises or yoga poses. Assessing your flexibility helps identify areas of tightness or limited range of motion, allowing you to incorporate specific stretching exercises to improve flexibility and prevent injuries.

4. Balance and Stability: Evaluating your balance and stability is crucial for preventing falls and injuries. It involves assessing your ability to maintain equilibrium and control your body's position during various movements. Balance exercises like standing on one leg or performing specific balance poses can help assess your stability. Identifying any balance issues can guide you in selecting appropriate balance exercises to improve stability and reduce the risk of falls.

5. Functional Movement: Assessing your functional movement involves evaluating your ability to perform everyday activities with ease and efficiency. It includes movements like bending, lifting, carrying, or reaching. Assessing your functional movement helps identify any limitations or asymmetries that may affect your daily activities or exercise performance. Addressing these limitations through targeted exercises can improve overall functional fitness.

By assessing your fitness level in these key areas, you can gain a comprehensive understanding of your current physical condition and capabilities. This self-assessment provides a baseline from which to track your progress as you incorporate weight-bearing exercises into your routine. It also helps you identify any specific areas that may require more attention or modifications during your exercise program.

Safety Considerations and Precautions

When starting a weight-bearing exercise program, it is crucial to prioritise safety to reduce the risk of injuries and ensure a positive exercise experience. Here are some important safety considerations and precautions to keep in mind:

1. Warm-Up and Cool-Down: Always begin your exercise session with a proper warm-up and end it with a cool-down. Warm-up exercises prepare your body for physical activity by increasing blood flow to the muscles and joints, loosening them up, and raising your body temperature. Cool-down exercises help gradually bring your heart rate and body temperature back to normal and prevent muscle soreness. Include dynamic stretches and light cardiovascular activities in your warm-up and cool-down routines.

2. Proper Form and Technique: Pay attention to your form and technique during weight-bearing exercises. Using correct form not only maximises the effectiveness of the exercises but also reduces the risk of injuries. If you are unsure about the proper form, consider working with a qualified fitness professional or exercise specialist who can guide you and provide feedback on your technique.

3. Gradual Progression: Start your weight-bearing exercise program at an appropriate intensity and gradually increase the duration, frequency, and intensity over time. This allows your body to adapt and reduces the risk of overuse injuries. Avoid pushing yourself too hard or progressing too quickly, as this can lead to burnout or injury. Listen to your body and give yourself enough time to recover between exercise sessions.

4. Use of Proper Equipment: Depending on the type of weight-bearing exercise you choose, it may be necessary to use proper equipment or gear. For example, if you are jogging or running, invest in a good pair of supportive and cushioned athletic shoes. If you are participating in high-impact activities like basketball or tennis, wear appropriate footwear and protective gear to minimise the risk of sprains or strains.

5. Stay Hydrated: Drink plenty of water before, during, and after your weight-bearing exercises to stay hydrated. Dehydration can negatively impact your performance and increase the risk of muscle cramps or fatigue. Aim to drink water regularly throughout the day, especially in warmer weather or during intense exercise sessions.

6. Listen to Your Body: Pay attention to your body's signals during exercise. If you experience pain, dizziness, or unusual discomfort, stop exercising and consult with your healthcare provider. It's normal to feel some muscle fatigue or mild soreness after exercise, but sharp or persistent pain may indicate an injury or overexertion.

7. *Modify Exercises as Needed:* If you have any physical limitations, joint issues, or injuries, modify the exercises to suit your needs. There are often alternative variations or adaptations available for different exercises that can reduce stress on certain areas of your body. Consult with a fitness professional or physical therapist for guidance on appropriate modifications.

8. *Consider Personal Safety:* If you are exercising outdoors, be mindful of your surroundings and ensure your safety. Choose well-lit areas, wear reflective clothing if exercising at night, and be aware of potential hazards or uneven surfaces. If participating in team sports or activities, follow the rules and guidelines to minimize the risk of collisions or accidents.

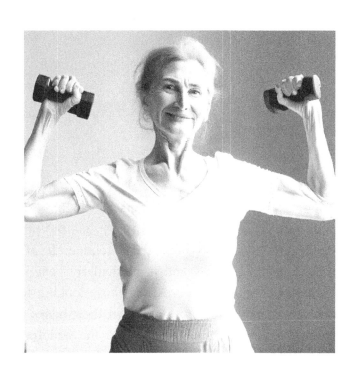

Chapter 4

Low-Impact
Weight-Bearing Exercises

Walking

Walking is a fantastic low-impact weight-bearing exercise that is accessible to almost everyone and can be easily incorporated into your daily routine. It offers numerous health benefits and is particularly beneficial for individuals with osteoporosis or those looking for a gentle yet effective way to strengthen their bones and improve overall fitness. Let's explore the benefits of walking and how to make the most out of this simple yet powerful exercise.

Benefits of Walking:

1. Bone Health: Walking is a weight-bearing exercise that puts stress on your bones, promoting bone density and strength. It helps stimulate the production of new bone tissue, which is crucial for individuals with osteoporosis. Regular walking can reduce the risk of fractures and improve overall bone health.

2. Cardiovascular Health: Walking is a great cardiovascular exercise that gets your heart pumping and improves circulation. It helps lower blood pressure, reduce the risk of heart disease, and improve overall cardiovascular fitness. Regular walking can also help manage weight, lower cholesterol levels, and improve insulin sensitivity.

3. Muscle Strength and Endurance: Walking engages various muscles, including those in your legs, hips, core, and arms if you swing them naturally while walking. It helps strengthen and tone these muscles, improving their endurance and overall functional strength.

4. Joint Health and Mobility: Walking is a low-impact exercise that puts minimal stress on your joints, making it suitable for individuals with joint issues or arthritis. It helps lubricate the joints, reduce stiffness, and improve joint mobility and flexibility.

5. Mental Well-being: Walking has numerous mental health benefits. It releases endorphins, the feel-good hormones that help reduce stress, anxiety, and depression. Walking outdoors in nature can have additional mood-boosting effects, providing a sense of tranquillity and improving overall mental well-being.

1. Start Slowly: If you're new to walking or have been sedentary for a while, start with shorter walks at a comfortable pace. Gradually increase your duration and intensity over time as your fitness level improves.

2. Maintain Proper Posture: Walk tall with your head up, shoulders relaxed, and abdominal muscles engaged. Swing your arms naturally and take smooth, comfortable strides. Focus on landing softly on your heels and rolling through your foot to push off with your toes.

3. Choose the Right Shoes: Invest in a good pair of supportive and cushioned walking shoes that fit well and provide proper arch support. This helps reduce the risk of foot or ankle discomfort and promotes a more comfortable walking experience.

4. Find Suitable Walking Surfaces: Opt for flat, even surfaces to minimise the risk of tripping or falling. Sidewalks, tracks, or well-maintained trails are ideal. If you prefer walking indoors, consider using a treadmill or walking track.

5. Gradually Increase Intensity: Once you've established a regular walking routine, challenge yourself by gradually increasing the intensity. This can include walking at a faster pace, incorporating intervals of brisk walking or adding gentle inclines to your route.

6. *Stay Consistent:* Aim for at least 30 minutes of moderate-intensity walking most days of the week. You can break it into smaller sessions if needed. Consistency is key to reaping the long-term benefits of walking.

Walking is a versatile and enjoyable low-impact weight-bearing exercise that can be customised to suit your fitness level and preferences. Whether you choose to walk alone, with a friend, or join a walking group, the key is to make it a regular part of your routine. Lace up your shoes, step outside, and let the benefits of walking enhance your bone health, cardiovascular fitness, and overall well-being.

Dancing

Dancing is a delightful and engaging form of exercise that combines movement, rhythm, and self-expression. Not only is it an enjoyable activity, but it also offers a range of health benefits, making it an excellent choice for low-impact weight-bearing exercise. Let's explore the world of dance and discover how it can contribute to strengthening your bones and improving your overall well-being.

Benefits of Dancing:

1. Bone Health: Dancing involves weight-bearing movements that put stress on your bones, stimulating bone growth and enhancing bone density. This is particularly beneficial for individuals with osteoporosis or those at risk of developing the condition. Regular dancing can help reduce the risk of fractures and improve skeletal strength.

2. Cardiovascular Fitness: Dancing is a fantastic cardiovascular workout that gets your heart pumping and increases endurance. It improves your cardiovascular health by elevating your heart rate, improving circulation, and enhancing lung capacity. Dancing helps to strengthen your heart and lowers the risk of cardiovascular diseases.

3. Muscle Strength and Endurance: Dancing engages various muscle groups, including your legs, core, arms, and back. As you move to the rhythm of the music, your muscles work to support your body and execute the dance steps. This helps to build strength, improve muscle tone, and enhance overall endurance.

4. Balance and Coordination: Dance requires coordination, balance, and body control. Through practising different dance styles, you can improve your balance and coordination skills, reducing the risk of falls and enhancing your overall stability.

5. Cognitive Benefits: Dancing is a mentally stimulating activity that involves learning and remembering dance routines, coordinating movements, and adapting to the rhythm and timing of the music. It can help enhance cognitive function, memory, and focus.

6. Emotional Well-being: Dancing is known for its positive impact on emotional well-being. It releases endorphins, the "feel-good" hormones, which can help reduce stress, anxiety, and depression. Dancing also provides a creative outlet for self-expression and can boost self-confidence and self-esteem.

Getting Started with Dancing:

1. Choose Your Style: There are various dance styles to explore, such as ballroom, salsa, hip-hop, jazz, or contemporary. Choose a style that resonates with you and matches your fitness level and interests. You can start with beginner-level classes or instructional videos.

2. Take Classes: Consider joining dance classes or workshops taught by qualified instructors. This will provide structured guidance and help you learn proper techniques and dance routines. Additionally, dancing in a group setting can add a social element to your exercise routine.

3. Dance at Home: If you prefer the comfort of your own home, there are many online dance tutorials and video resources available. You can follow along with instructional videos or dance to your favorite music. Clear a space to ensure you have enough room to move freely and safely.

4. Start Slowly: If you're new to dancing or have been inactive for a while, start with shorter sessions and gradually increase the duration and intensity. Allow your body to adapt and progress at a pace that feels comfortable for you.

5. *Warm-up and Cool-down:* Prior to dancing, warm up your body with dynamic stretches and movements to prepare your muscles and joints. After your dance session, cool down with gentle stretches to improve flexibility and prevent muscle soreness.

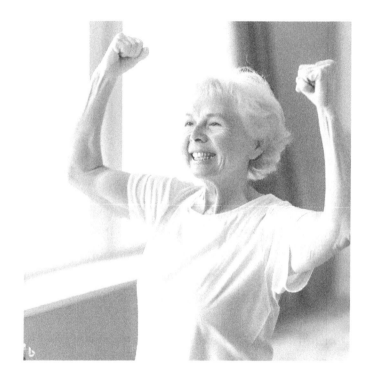

Water Aerobics

Water aerobics, also known as aqua aerobics or water exercise, is a fantastic low-impact workout that takes place in the water. It combines cardiovascular exercise, strength training, and flexibility movements to provide a comprehensive fitness routine while minimising stress on your joints. Let's dive into the refreshing world of water aerobics and explore its benefits for your bone health and overall well-being.

Benefits of Water Aerobics:

1. Low-Impact Exercise: Water aerobics is performed in a pool, where the buoyancy of water reduces the impact on your joints. This makes it an ideal choice for individuals with arthritis, joint pain, or those recovering from injuries. The water's buoyancy supports your body, making you feel lighter and allowing for fluid movements without straining your joints.

2. Cardiovascular Fitness: Water aerobics is a great way to improve cardiovascular health and build endurance. The water provides resistance to your movements, making your heart work harder to pump blood and oxygen throughout your body. Regular water aerobics sessions can help strengthen your heart, lower blood pressure, and improve overall cardiovascular fitness.

3. Muscle Strength and Tone: The resistance provided by the water acts as a natural form of resistance training, challenging your muscles and improving their strength and endurance. As you move through the water, your muscles work against the resistance, targeting various muscle groups including your arms, legs, core, and back. Water aerobics can help tone your muscles, increase lean muscle mass, and improve overall body strength.

4. Joint Flexibility and Range of Motion: Exercising in water allows for greater freedom of movement and can help improve joint flexibility and range of motion. The water's buoyancy supports your joints, reducing the stress and pressure on them. This is particularly beneficial for individuals with arthritis or stiffness in their joints.

5. Balance and Coordination: Water aerobics challenges your balance and coordination skills as you perform various movements in an aquatic environment. The water's resistance forces you to engage your core muscles and maintain stability. Regular participation in water aerobics can enhance your balance, coordination, and overall body awareness.

Getting Started with Water Aerobics:

1. Find a Pool: Look for a local swimming pool or fitness center that offers water aerobics classes or open swim sessions. Make sure the water is warm enough for your comfort.

2. Join a Class: Consider participating in a water aerobics class led by a qualified instructor. These classes are designed to provide a structured workout with guidance on proper techniques and exercises suitable for different fitness levels.

3. Warm-up and Stretch: Before starting your water aerobics session, perform a warm-up routine that includes gentle movements and stretches to prepare your body for exercise.

4. Choose the Right Equipment: Depending on the class or your personal preference, you may need specific equipment such as water dumbbells, foam noodles, or resistance bands. These tools can add variety and intensity to your workouts.

5. Stay Hydrated: Even though you're in the water, it's important to stay hydrated. Drink water before, during, and after your water aerobics session to keep your body properly hydrated.

6. *Listen to Your Body:* Pay attention to how your body feels during the exercises. If any movement causes pain or discomfort, modify or avoid it. It's essential to work within your own comfort zone and gradually increase the intensity as you become more conditioned.

Water aerobics provides a refreshing and enjoyable way to engage in low-impact weight-bearing exercise. It offers a multitude of benefits for individuals of all fitness levels, including those with joint issues or mobility limitations. Whether you're looking to improve cardiovascular fitness, strengthen your muscles, or enhance flexibility, water aerobics can be a fantastic addition to your exercise routine.

Tai Chi

Tai Chi is an ancient Chinese martial art that combines slow, flowing movements with deep breathing and mindfulness. It is widely practised for its numerous health benefits and is particularly suitable as a low-impact weight-bearing exercise. Let's delve into the graceful world of Tai Chi and discover how it can strengthen your bones, improve balance, and promote overall well-being.

Benefits of Tai Chi:

1. Balance and Stability: Tai Chi incorporates a series of deliberate, controlled movements that require shifting your weight from one leg to another while maintaining proper posture. This focus on weight transfer and body alignment helps improve balance and stability, reducing the risk of falls and related injuries.

2. Bone Health: While Tai Chi is considered a low-impact exercise, it still provides weight-bearing benefits for your bones. The gentle weight shifts and movements during Tai Chi stimulate bone cells, encouraging bone growth and density. Regular practice of Tai Chi can help slow down bone loss and promote skeletal strength.

3. Flexibility and Range of Motion: Tai Chi involves gentle stretches and fluid movements that help improve flexibility and increase the range of motion in your joints. The slow, controlled motions allow you to gradually stretch and lengthen your muscles, promoting suppleness and reducing muscle stiffness.

4. Muscle Strength: Despite its slow pace, Tai Chi engages various muscle groups throughout the body. As you perform the movements, you activate and strengthen your legs, arms, core, and back muscles. Improved muscle strength not only enhances physical performance but also provides better support for your bones and joints.

5. Stress Reduction and Mindfulness: Tai Chi emphasises deep, relaxed breathing and focused attention on the present moment. This meditative aspect of the practice promotes relaxation, reduces stress, and cultivates mindfulness. The gentle, flowing movements combined with breathing techniques create a harmonious mind-body connection, promoting a sense of calm and well-being.

1. Find an Instructor or Class: Look for a qualified Tai Chi instructor or local classes in your community. Learning Tai Chi from an experienced teacher ensures proper technique and guidance as you begin your practice.

2. Choose Appropriate Attire: Wear loose, comfortable clothing and flat shoes that provide stability and allow for ease of movement. Avoid restrictive clothing that may hinder your range of motion.

3. Warm-up and Cool-down: Begin each Tai Chi session with a warm-up routine, which may include gentle stretches and loosening exercises to prepare your body for the movements. Afterward, cool down with relaxing, deep breathing and gentle movements.

4. Start with Basic Movements: Beginners typically start with learning a few basic Tai Chi movements or forms. These forms consist of a series of connected postures performed in a slow, continuous manner. Practice and gradually add more movements as you become familiar with the basics.

5. Practice Regularly: Consistency is key when practising Tai Chi. Aim for regular practice sessions, gradually increasing the duration and frequency as you progress. Even short daily practice sessions can yield benefits for your physical and mental well-being.

6. *Listen to Your Body:* Tai Chi should be practised at your own pace and comfort level. Pay attention to your body's feedback and avoid pushing beyond your limits. Modify the movements if needed and focus on maintaining proper alignment and relaxation throughout your practice.

Tai Chi offers a gentle yet powerful approach to low-impact weight-bearing exercise. Its fluid movements, deep breathing, and meditative aspects contribute to overall physical and mental wellness. As we continue exploring the realm of low-impact weight-bearing exercises, we will uncover the benefits of yoga and its potential impact on bone health and flexibility. Let's continue on our path to stronger bones and a healthier lifestyle through the practice of these mindful exercises.

Yoga

Yoga is an ancient practice originating from India that combines physical postures, breathing exercises, meditation, and relaxation techniques. It has gained popularity worldwide for its holistic approach to health and well-being. While often known for its flexibility benefits, yoga also offers low-impact weight-bearing exercises that can contribute to strengthening your bones and improving overall fitness. Let's explore the transformative world of yoga and its potential impact on your bone health.

Benefits of Yoga:

1. Strength and Stability: Yoga poses, also known as asanas, require the engagement of various muscle groups, promoting overall strength and stability. Weight-bearing poses such as standing poses, balances, and certain variations of inversions provide the necessary stimulus to strengthen your bones and muscles.

2. Bone Health: Yoga postures that involve weight-bearing on your arms, legs, or spine can help improve bone density. The gentle stress applied to the bones during yoga practice stimulates bone-building cells, contributing to better skeletal strength and reduced risk of osteoporosis-related fractures.

3. Flexibility and Range of Motion: Yoga incorporates a wide range of movements and stretches that improve flexibility and increase the range of motion in your joints. Regular practice can help alleviate stiffness, increase joint mobility, and enhance overall physical performance.

4. Balance and Coordination: Many yoga poses require balance and focus, challenging your coordination skills. Through regular practice, you can improve your balance, proprioception (awareness of your body in space), and coordination, leading to better stability and a reduced risk of falls.

5. Stress Reduction and Mind-Body Connection: Yoga is well-known for its calming effects on the mind and body. The combination of breath awareness, mindfulness, and physical movement cultivates a sense of relaxation, reduces stress, and enhances overall well-being. By reducing stress, yoga indirectly supports bone health, as chronic stress can negatively impact bone density.

Getting Started with Yoga:

1. Choose a Yoga Style: There are various styles of yoga, each with its own emphasis and intensity level. Some popular styles include Hatha, Vinyasa, Iyengar, and Restorative. Explore different styles and find one that aligns with your goals and preferences.

2. Find a Qualified Instructor or Online Resources: It is recommended to learn yoga from a qualified instructor, especially if you are new to the practice. Look for local yoga studios, community centers, or online platforms that offer beginner-friendly classes led by experienced teachers.

3. Start with Beginner-friendly Poses: Begin your yoga journey with basic poses suitable for beginners. These poses focus on building foundational strength, flexibility, and body awareness. Common beginner poses include Mountain Pose (Tadasana), Warrior Poses (Virabhadrasana), and Downward-Facing Dog (Adho Mukha Svanasana).

4. Practise Mindful Breathing: Breath awareness is an essential aspect of yoga. Learn and practise different breathing techniques, such as deep belly breathing (Diaphragmatic breathing) or alternate nostril breathing (Nadi Shodhana), to enhance relaxation and focus during your yoga practice.

5. *Listen to Your Body:* Yoga is a practice of self-awareness and self-care. Pay attention to your body's signals and avoid pushing yourself beyond your limits. Honour your body's capabilities and modify or skip poses that feel uncomfortable or cause pain. Yoga is meant to be a gentle and nurturing practice.

6. *Consistency and Progression:* Consistent practice is key to reaping the benefits of yoga. Start with shorter sessions and gradually increase the duration and frequency as your body adapts. Even a few minutes of daily practice can make a difference in your strength, flexibility, and overall well-being.

Yoga offers a holistic approach to low-impact weight-bearing exercise, combining physical postures, breathwork, and mindfulness. As we continue our exploration of low-impact weight-bearing exercises, we will uncover the benefits of strength-training exercises and their role in maintaining bone health. Let's continue on our path to stronger bones and a healthier lifestyle through the practice of these mindful exercises.

Chapter 5

High-Impact Weight-Bearing Exercises

Jogging

Jogging, a form of running at a relaxed and steady pace, is an excellent high-impact weight-bearing exercise that can contribute to your bone health and overall fitness. Whether you're a seasoned runner or just starting out, jogging offers numerous benefits that go beyond cardiovascular endurance. In this section, we will explore the advantages of jogging and how to incorporate it into your exercise routine effectively.

Benefits of Jogging:

1. Bone Health: Jogging is a weight-bearing exercise that puts stress on your bones, stimulating them to become stronger and denser. The repetitive impact of jogging helps build and maintain bone mass, reducing the risk of osteoporosis and fractures. It specifically targets the weight-bearing bones of your legs, hips, and spine, making it a beneficial exercise for these areas.

2. Cardiovascular Fitness: Jogging is an effective way to improve cardiovascular endurance. Regular jogging sessions increase your heart rate, improve blood circulation, and enhance lung capacity. This leads to a stronger cardiovascular system, increased stamina, and improved overall fitness.

3. Muscle Strength and Endurance: Jogging engages multiple muscle groups, including your quadriceps, hamstrings, calves, and glutes. These muscles work together to propel your body forward, providing strength and endurance benefits. Regular jogging can tone and strengthen these muscles, improving your overall lower body strength.

4. Weight Management: Jogging is an effective exercise for burning calories and maintaining a healthy weight. It can help you shed excess pounds and maintain a balanced body composition. Regular jogging sessions, combined with a healthy diet, can contribute to weight management and overall well-being.

5. Mental Health and Stress Relief: Jogging is not only beneficial for your physical health but also for your mental well-being. Engaging in regular jogging can help reduce stress levels, alleviate anxiety and depression, and improve your mood. The release of endorphins during exercise creates a sense of well-being and boosts mental clarity.

Getting Started with Jogging:

1. Consult with Your Healthcare Provider: If you are new to jogging or have any underlying health conditions, it is essential to consult with your healthcare provider before starting a jogging routine. They can provide guidance based on your individual circumstances and ensure that jogging is safe for you.

2. Proper Warm-up and Cool-down: Before each jogging session, warm up your body with dynamic stretches, such as leg swings, hip circles, and walking lunges. This helps prepare your muscles, joints, and cardiovascular system for the activity. After jogging, cool down with gentle stretches to prevent muscle soreness and aid in recovery.

3. Gradual Progression: If you are new to jogging or returning after a break, start with a manageable pace and distance. Gradually increase the intensity and duration of your jogging sessions over time. Listen to your body and give yourself ample time to adapt and build endurance.

4. Proper Form and Technique: Focus on maintaining good posture while jogging. Keep your head up, shoulders relaxed, and core engaged. Land with a mid-foot strike, allowing your foot to roll naturally from heel to toe. Avoid overstriding, which can put excess stress on your joints.

5. *Choose Suitable Footwear:* Invest in a pair of well-fitting running shoes that provide adequate support and cushioning. Proper footwear can help prevent injuries and enhance your comfort while jogging. Visit a specialised running store to get fitted for the right shoes based on your foot type and running style.

6. *Listen to Your Body:* Pay attention to any signs of discomfort or pain while jogging. If you experience persistent pain, reduce your intensity or take a break to allow for recovery. It's important to strike a balance between pushing your limits and respecting your body's needs.

Jogging can be a rewarding high-impact weight-bearing exercise that strengthens your bones, improves your cardiovascular fitness, and enhances your overall well-being. By incorporating jogging into your exercise routine and following the guidelines mentioned above, you can reap the numerous benefits it offers. Lace up your running shoes, hit the pavement, and enjoy the exhilarating experience of jogging while promoting your bone health and overall fitness.

Jumping Rope

Jumping rope, a classic childhood activity, is not only a fun pastime but also a fantastic high-impact weight-bearing exercise that can strengthen your bones and boost your cardiovascular fitness. It offers a wide range of benefits, including improved coordination, agility, and endurance. In this section, we will explore the advantages of jumping rope and how to incorporate it into your exercise routine effectively.

Benefits of Jumping Rope:

1. Bone Health: Jumping rope is a weight-bearing exercise that subjects your bones to impact forces, which stimulates the production of new bone tissue. This, in turn, strengthens your bones, increases bone density, and reduces the risk of osteoporosis and fractures. It primarily targets the bones of your legs and hips, making it an excellent exercise for these areas.

2. Cardiovascular Endurance: Jumping rope is a highly effective aerobic exercise that elevates your heart rate, improving cardiovascular endurance. It increases the efficiency of your heart and lungs, enhances blood circulation, and helps you develop better stamina and overall fitness.

3. Full-Body Workout: Jumping rope engages multiple muscle groups, including your calves, thighs, glutes, shoulders, and core. The continuous jumping motion works these muscles in a coordinated manner, providing a comprehensive full-body workout. Regular jump rope sessions can help tone and strengthen these muscles, enhancing your overall strength and stability.

4. Coordination and Agility: Jumping rope requires precise coordination between your hands and feet, improving your motor skills and hand-eye coordination. The rhythmic nature of the exercise also enhances your agility, balance, and spatial awareness. These benefits extend beyond your exercise routine and can positively impact your daily activities and sports performance.

5. Calorie Burning and Weight Management: Jumping rope is a highly efficient calorie-burning exercise. It can help you shed excess pounds, improve body composition, and support weight management. The intensity of jumping rope allows you to burn a significant number of calories in a relatively short amount of time.

1. Select the Right Rope: Choose a jump rope that is appropriate for your height and fitness level. The rope should be long enough to comfortably clear over your head and allow for smooth rotations. Consider using a lightweight and adjustable rope to suit your preferences.

2. Find a Suitable Surface: Jumping rope is most effective when performed on a flat, cushioned surface. Opt for a shock-absorbing surface such as a gym mat or a forgiving outdoor surface like grass or a rubberized track. Avoid concrete or hard surfaces that may cause excessive impact on your joints.

3. Warm-Up and Cool-Down: Prior to jumping rope, warm up your body with dynamic stretches or light aerobic exercises to prepare your muscles and joints for the activity. After your workout, cool down with gentle stretches to promote muscle recovery and prevent tightness.

4. Start with Basic Jumps: Begin by mastering the basic jump, also known as the "two-foot jump." Stand with your feet together, holding the rope handles. Swing the rope over your head and jump over it, clearing the rope with both feet at the same time. Focus on maintaining a relaxed but engaged posture and a consistent rhythm.

5. Progress to Variations: Once you feel comfortable with the basic jump, you can explore different variations to challenge yourself further. Try single-leg jumps, alternating foot jumps, high knees, or double unders (two rotations of the rope per jump) to add variety and intensity to your workout.

6. Gradual Progression: Start with shorter jump rope sessions and gradually increase the duration as your fitness level improves. Listen to your body and gradually increase the intensity and speed of your jumps over time. Remember to take breaks and pace yourself to avoid overexertion.

7. Maintain Proper Form: Keep an upright posture, with your chest lifted and your shoulders relaxed. Land softly on the balls of your feet, allowing your knees to flex slightly to absorb the impact. Maintain a consistent rhythm and avoid excessive tension in your arms and shoulders.

8. Include Jump Rope in Your Routine: Incorporate jump rope sessions into your weekly exercise routine. Aim for at least 10-15 minutes of continuous jumping or shorter intervals with rest periods in between. You can gradually increase the duration as your fitness improves.

Jumping rope is a versatile and effective high-impact weight-bearing exercise that can improve your bone health, cardiovascular fitness, coordination, and overall strength. By following the guidelines outlined above and incorporating jumping rope into your fitness regimen, you can experience the numerous benefits it offers while enjoying a fun and challenging workout. Grab your jump rope, find your rhythm, and leap into better health and fitness.

Tennis

Tennis is not only a popular and engaging sport but also an excellent high-impact weight-bearing exercise that can benefit your bone health, cardiovascular fitness, and overall strength. It offers a dynamic combination of physical activity, strategic thinking, and social interaction. In this section, we will explore the advantages of playing tennis and how to incorporate it into your exercise routine effectively.

Benefits of Tennis:

1. Bone Health: Tennis involves a variety of weight-bearing movements, such as running, jumping, and pivoting, which place stress on your bones. This impact stimulates your bones to become stronger, denser, and more resilient. Regular participation in tennis can help improve bone density and reduce the risk of osteoporosis and fractures, particularly in weight-bearing bones like the legs, hips, and spine.

2. Cardiovascular Fitness: Tennis is a fast-paced sport that requires continuous movement and bursts of intense effort. Playing tennis can significantly improve your cardiovascular endurance, as it elevates your heart rate, enhances lung capacity, and improves overall cardiovascular health. The combination of aerobic and anaerobic elements in tennis helps strengthen your heart and lungs, leading to increased stamina and improved fitness levels.

*3. **Muscle Strength and Endurance:*** Tennis engages multiple muscle groups throughout your body. The repetitive swinging of the racket strengthens your arm, shoulder, and back muscles, while the quick lateral movements and lunges engage your leg muscles. Regular participation in tennis can improve muscular strength, endurance, and overall body tone.

*4. **Agility and Coordination:*** Tennis requires quick reflexes, agility, and hand-eye coordination. The sport involves rapid changes in direction, split-second decision-making, and precise shot placement. These aspects of tennis enhance your agility, balance, coordination, and spatial awareness, which can be beneficial in various daily activities and sports.

*5. **Mental Benefits:*** Tennis is a mentally stimulating sport that challenges your strategic thinking, focus, and concentration. It promotes improved mental agility, problem-solving skills, and quick decision-making. Engaging in tennis can help reduce stress, boost mood, and enhance overall cognitive function.

Getting Started with Tennis:

1. Learn the Basics: If you are new to tennis, consider taking lessons from a qualified instructor or joining a beginner's group. Learning the fundamental techniques, rules, and strategies of tennis will help you enjoy the sport while minimising the risk of injury.

2. Gear and Equipment: Start with a proper tennis racket that suits your grip size and skill level. Choose tennis shoes that provide good support, cushioning, and traction to prevent foot and ankle injuries. Wear comfortable and breathable clothing suitable for outdoor or indoor play, depending on the tennis court you use.

3. Warm-Up and Stretching: Prior to playing tennis, warm up your body with a light jog or brisk walk to increase blood flow and raise your body temperature. Perform dynamic stretches that target the muscles involved in tennis, such as shoulder circles, lunges, side shuffles, and arm swings. This helps prepare your muscles, joints, and cardiovascular system for the activity.

4. Start Slowly: Begin with shorter practice sessions and gradually increase the duration and intensity as your fitness level improves. Focus on developing proper technique and footwork before playing more competitive matches.

5. Proper Footwork and Movement: Tennis requires efficient footwork and quick changes in direction. Practise proper footwork techniques, such as split steps, side steps, and pivots, to improve your agility and court coverage. Maintain a balanced and athletic stance, with your knees slightly bent and ready to move in any direction.

6. Play with Others: Tennis is a social sport that can be enjoyed with friends, family members, or at local tennis clubs. Engaging in friendly matches or joining leagues can add excitement and motivation to your tennis practice. It also provides an opportunity for social interaction and friendly competition.

Remember to listen to your body, stay hydrated, and rest when needed. Tennis can be physically demanding, so pace yourself and gradually increase your playing time and intensity as your fitness improves. Enjoy the exhilaration of the game while reaping the numerous health benefits that tennis offers.

Basketball

Basketball is a dynamic and fast-paced sport that not only provides excitement and entertainment but also offers a range of health benefits. It is a high-impact weight-bearing exercise that can improve your bone health, cardiovascular fitness, strength, and coordination. In this section, we will explore the advantages of playing basketball and how to incorporate it into your exercise routine effectively.

Benefits of Basketball:

1. Bone Health: Playing basketball involves running, jumping, and quick changes in direction, which place stress on your bones. This weight-bearing impact stimulates bone growth and strength, helping to improve bone density and reduce the risk of osteoporosis and fractures. The multidirectional movements of basketball also help strengthen the bones of your legs, hips, and spine.

2. Cardiovascular Fitness: Basketball is an intense aerobic activity that requires constant movement, sprinting, and endurance. The fast-paced nature of the game elevates your heart rate, improves blood circulation, and enhances cardiovascular endurance. Regular participation in basketball can improve your lung capacity, strengthen your heart, and boost overall cardiovascular fitness.

3. *Muscle Strength and Endurance:* Basketball involves various physical demands that engage multiple muscle groups. Dribbling, shooting, and passing work your arm, shoulder, and core muscles, while running and jumping engage your leg muscles. The continuous movement and quick bursts of power in basketball contribute to improved muscular strength, endurance, and overall body toning.

4. *Coordination and Agility:* Basketball requires precise hand-eye coordination, quick reflexes, and agile footwork. Dribbling, passing, and shooting the ball demand coordination between your hands and eyes, while defending and maneuvering on the court require quick changes in direction and balance. Regular basketball play enhances your agility, balance, coordination, and spatial awareness.

5. *Teamwork and Social Interaction:* Basketball is often played in a team setting, fostering camaraderie, cooperation, and communication. Joining a basketball team or playing pickup games with friends can provide social interaction and a sense of belonging. The teamwork and strategic elements of basketball not only improve your physical fitness but also contribute to your mental well-being.

1. Learn the Basics: If you are new to basketball, familiarise yourself with the rules, basic techniques, and positions of the game. Consider taking lessons or participating in beginner programs to develop the necessary skills and understanding.

2. Gear and Equipment: Wear appropriate basketball shoes that provide good support, cushioning, and traction to prevent foot and ankle injuries. Choose comfortable and breathable clothing that allows for freedom of movement. Carry a properly inflated basketball to practice shooting, dribbling, and passing.

3. Warm-Up and Stretching: Prior to playing basketball, warm up your body with light aerobic exercises like jogging or jumping jacks to increase blood flow and warm up your muscles. Perform dynamic stretches that target the muscles involved in basketball, such as leg swings, arm circles, and torso rotations. This helps prepare your muscles, joints, and cardiovascular system for the activity.

4. Start with Skill Development: Focus on developing fundamental basketball skills, such as shooting, dribbling, passing, and basic footwork. Practice these skills individually or with a partner before engaging in game situations. Improving your technique and coordination will enhance your overall performance and enjoyment of the sport.

5. Find a Court and Play: Locate a basketball court in your community or join a local league or pickup game. Engage in friendly matches, participate in organized competitions, or simply shoot hoops with friends. Regular basketball play will allow you to further refine your skills, build endurance, and experience the exhilaration of the game.

6. Stay Safe and Hydrated: Protect yourself from injuries by using proper techniques, wearing protective gear like knee pads or ankle braces if necessary, and listening to your body. Stay hydrated by drinking plenty of water before, during, and after playing basketball to maintain optimal performance and prevent dehydration.

Hiking

Hiking is an enjoyable and accessible outdoor activity that offers a range of health benefits while allowing you to connect with nature. It is a high-impact weight-bearing exercise that engages your muscles, promotes cardiovascular fitness, and provides a refreshing escape from the urban environment. In this section, we will explore the advantages of hiking and how to make the most of this invigorating exercise.

Benefits of Hiking:

1. Bone Health: Hiking involves walking over varied terrain, which places stress on your bones and promotes bone strength and density. The weight-bearing nature of hiking helps to improve bone health, reduce the risk of osteoporosis, and enhance overall skeletal strength. The uneven surfaces encountered during hikes also engage the smaller stabilising muscles around your joints, contributing to better joint stability.

2. Cardiovascular Fitness: Hiking is a form of aerobic exercise that gets your heart pumping and improves cardiovascular fitness. Walking uphill, navigating uneven terrain, and maintaining a consistent pace during a hike elevate your heart rate and enhance blood circulation. Regular hiking can strengthen your heart, lower blood pressure, and improve lung capacity.

*3. **Muscular Strength and Endurance:*** Hiking engages the muscles of your lower body, including your quadriceps, hamstrings, glutes, and calves. Uphill climbs and descents require additional effort, helping to build muscular strength and endurance in these muscle groups. Additionally, carrying a backpack while hiking can further challenge your muscles and contribute to overall body toning.

*4. **Weight Management:*** Hiking is an effective exercise for weight management and burning calories. The varying intensity and duration of hikes allow you to customise your workout according to your fitness level and goals. Regular hiking can contribute to calorie expenditure, promote fat loss, and help maintain a healthy body weight.

*5. **Mental Well-being:*** Spending time in nature and engaging in physical activity have been linked to numerous mental health benefits. Hiking provides an opportunity to unplug from daily stressors, enjoy the beauty of the natural environment, and boost your mood. The combination of fresh air, natural surroundings, and physical exertion during hikes can reduce anxiety, alleviate symptoms of depression, and enhance overall mental well-being.

Getting Started with Hiking:

1. Choose Suitable Trails: Start with hiking trails that match your fitness level and experience. Consider factors such as trail length, elevation gain, and terrain difficulty. Begin with shorter, less challenging hikes and gradually progress to more advanced trails as your fitness improves.

2. Gear and Equipment: Wear comfortable and supportive hiking shoes or boots that provide stability and protect your feet from rough terrain. Dress in layers to accommodate changing weather conditions and pack essential items such as a backpack, water bottle, map, compass, sunscreen, insect repellent, and snacks. Consider using trekking poles for added stability and reduced impact on your joints.

3. Warm-Up and Stretching: Before starting a hike, perform a warm-up routine that includes light cardio exercises such as walking or gentle stretching to prepare your muscles for the activity. Focus on stretching your legs, hips, and lower back to enhance flexibility and reduce the risk of injuries.

4. *Hydration and Nutrition:* Stay hydrated by drinking water before, during, and after your hike. Pack sufficient water and hydrating snacks to replenish electrolytes and energy during longer hikes. Additionally, carry nutritious snacks such as trail mix, energy bars, or fruits to sustain your energy levels throughout the hike.

5. *Start Slow and Gradually Increase Difficulty:* Begin with shorter, easier hikes to acclimate your body to the physical demands of hiking. As your fitness improves, gradually increase the duration, distance, and difficulty level of your hikes. Challenge yourself by tackling more challenging terrains or longer distances to further enhance your fitness and endurance.

6. *Safety Considerations:* Prioritise your safety by familiarising yourself with the trail maps, following marked trails, and informing someone about your hiking plans. Be aware of weather conditions and dress accordingly. Practice Leave No Trace principles by respecting nature, avoiding littering, and staying on designated trails.

Hiking provides an opportunity to explore nature, improve your physical fitness, and enjoy the many benefits of being outdoors. By incorporating hiking into your exercise routine, you can enhance your bone health, cardiovascular fitness, muscular strength, and mental well-being. Lace up your hiking boots, find a scenic trail, and embark on an adventure that nourishes both your body and soul.

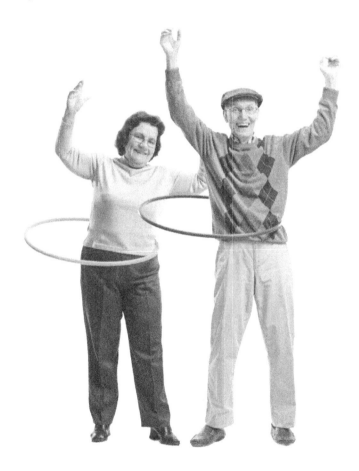

Chapter 6

Strength-Training Exercises

Bicep Curls

Strength training exercises are essential for building and maintaining strong muscles, improving bone density, and enhancing overall physical fitness. In this chapter, we will delve into various strength-training exercises that target different muscle groups. Let's begin with one of the most popular exercises for the arms: bicep curls.

Bicep curls specifically target the bicep muscles located in the front of your upper arms. By performing bicep curls regularly, you can strengthen and tone these muscles, enhancing both their functional and aesthetic appeal.

Here's how to perform bicep curls correctly:

1. Stand upright with your feet shoulder-width apart and your knees slightly bent. Hold a dumbbell in each hand with your palms facing forward. Alternatively, you can

use resistance bands or other weightlifting equipment if available.

2. Keep your upper arms close to your sides and your elbows tucked in. This is the starting position for the exercise.

3. Slowly exhale as you bend your elbows and lift the weights toward your shoulders, contracting your biceps. Maintain a controlled and steady motion throughout the movement. It's important to avoid using momentum or swinging the weights.

4. Pause for a moment when the weights are at shoulder level, and squeeze your biceps.

5. Inhale as you gradually lower the weights back to the starting position, fully extending your arms. This completes one repetition.

6. Repeat the exercise for the desired number of repetitions, typically 8 to 12, depending on your fitness level and goals.

Tips for Performing Bicep Curls:

- Start with lighter weights and gradually increase the resistance as your muscles become stronger.
- Maintain proper form throughout the exercise, keeping your back straight and avoiding excessive swinging or arching of the back.
- Focus on the contraction of your bicep muscles during the upward phase of the movement and control the descent to maximise the benefits.
- Breathe steadily throughout the exercise, exhaling during the exertion phase and inhaling during the lowering phase.
- If you experience any pain or discomfort, reduce the weight or consult with a fitness professional to ensure proper technique and form.

Benefits of Bicep Curls:

- Increased Muscle Strength: Bicep curls help strengthen the bicep muscles, improving their ability to perform daily tasks involving lifting or pulling.
- Enhanced Upper Body Function: Strong biceps contribute to better upper body strength and functionality, benefiting activities like carrying groceries, lifting objects, or performing sports-related movements.

- Improved Muscle Tone: Regularly performing bicep curls can help tone and define the appearance of your arms, giving them a more sculpted and athletic look.
- Increased Bone Density: Strength training exercises like bicep curls stimulate bone growth, which can help maintain and improve bone density, reducing the risk of osteoporosis.
- Overall Metabolic Boost: Strength training exercises, including bicep curls, contribute to an increased metabolic rate, aiding in weight management and overall calorie burning.

Incorporating bicep curls into your strength-training routine can provide significant benefits to your arm muscles, upper body strength, and bone health. Combine them with other exercises targeting different muscle groups for a well-rounded strength-training program. Remember to prioritise proper form, gradually increase the intensity, and listen to your body to ensure safe and effective workouts.

Squats

Squats are a fundamental strength-training exercise that targets multiple muscle groups, primarily the quadriceps, hamstrings, and glutes. They are highly effective for building lower body strength, improving balance, and enhancing overall functional fitness. In this section, we will explore the proper technique and benefits of squats.

How to Perform Squats:

1. Stand with your feet slightly wider than shoulder-width apart, toes pointing forward or slightly outward. Keep your spine neutral, chest lifted, and shoulders relaxed.

2. Engage your core muscles by drawing your navel in toward your spine. This will help stabilize your torso throughout the exercise.

3. Begin the squat movement by bending at your knees and hips, as if you're sitting back into an imaginary chair. Keep your weight distributed evenly through your feet and heels firmly planted on the ground.

4. Lower your body down until your thighs are parallel to the ground, or as close to parallel as you can

comfortably manage. Ensure that your knees are tracking in line with your toes and not collapsing inward.

5. Maintain a controlled descent, then exhale and push through your heels to return to the starting position, fully extending your hips and knees. This completes one repetition.

6. Repeat the movement for the desired number of repetitions, typically 8 to 12, depending on your fitness level and goals.

Tips for Performing Squats:

- Keep your chest lifted and gaze forward to maintain proper spinal alignment.
- Avoid rounding your lower back or allowing your knees to extend past your toes during the squat. This can place excessive stress on your joints.
- Engage your glute muscles as you return to the starting position to maximize the benefits of the exercise.
- Start with bodyweight squats or use a weight that is comfortable for you. As you become stronger and more confident, you can gradually increase the resistance by using dumbbells, barbells, or kettlebells.
- If you have any knee or joint issues, it's advisable to consult with a healthcare professional or a qualified

fitness trainer to ensure proper form and modifications, if needed.

- Lower Body Strength: Squats target the muscles of the lower body, including the quadriceps, hamstrings, glutes, and calves. By regularly performing squats, you can strengthen these muscles, improving your ability to perform everyday activities such as walking, climbing stairs, or lifting objects.
- Functional Fitness: Squats mimic movements used in daily life, making them highly functional. The strength and stability developed through squats can enhance your balance, coordination, and overall physical performance.
- Bone Health: Squats are weight-bearing exercises that stimulate bone growth and density, reducing the risk of osteoporosis and promoting strong and healthy bones.
- Calorie Burning: Squats engage large muscle groups, which helps to increase calorie expenditure and support weight management goals.
- Core Stability: Squats require activation of the core muscles to maintain balance and stability throughout the movement. Regular squatting can contribute to a stronger and more stable core.

Lunges

Lunges are a highly effective strength-training exercise that primarily targets the muscles of the lower body, including the quadriceps, hamstrings, glutes, and calves. They are a versatile exercise that can be performed with or without weights and offer numerous benefits for building lower body strength, improving balance, and enhancing functional fitness. In this section, we will explore the proper technique and benefits of lunges.

How to Perform Lunges:

1. Stand tall with your feet hip-width apart and your hands on your hips or relaxed at your sides.

2. Take a step forward with your right foot, ensuring that your feet are hip-width apart and your toes are pointing forward.

3. Lower your body by bending your knees until your front thigh is parallel to the ground, and your back knee is hovering just above the floor. Keep your torso upright and engage your core for stability.

4. Ensure that your front knee is directly above your ankle, and your back knee is positioned underneath your hip.

5. Push through your front heel to return to the starting position, fully extending your front knee and hip. This completes one repetition.

6. Repeat the movement with your left leg, stepping forward and lunging, following the same technique.

Tips for Performing Lunges:

- Maintain proper posture throughout the exercise by keeping your chest lifted, shoulders relaxed, and gaze forward.
- Engage your core muscles to stabilize your body during the lunge.
- Keep your front knee in line with your toes, avoiding it from collapsing inward.
- Take a long enough step forward to create a 90-degree angle with your front knee when lowered into the lunge position.
- Start with bodyweight lunges or use dumbbells or other weighted objects to add resistance as your strength increases.
- If you have knee or joint issues, it's advisable to consult with a healthcare professional or a qualified fitness trainer to ensure proper form and modifications, if needed.

Benefits of Lunges:

- Lower Body Strength: Lunges target the muscles of the lower body, including the quadriceps, hamstrings, glutes, and calves. By incorporating lunges into your exercise routine, you can strengthen and tone these muscles, improving your overall lower body strength.
- Balance and Stability: Lunges require coordination and balance, which help enhance stability and proprioception.
- Functional Movement: Lunges mimic movements used in daily life, such as walking, climbing stairs, or getting up from a chair. By performing lunges, you can improve your ability to perform these functional movements with ease and efficiency.
- Core Engagement: Lunges engage the core muscles to maintain balance and stability during the exercise, contributing to a stronger and more stable core.
- Flexibility and Range of Motion: Lunges promote hip flexibility and improve the range of motion in the lower body joints, enhancing overall mobility.

Push-Ups

Push-ups are a classic and highly effective strength-training exercise that primarily targets the muscles of the upper body, including the chest, shoulders, triceps, and core. They are a compound exercise that engages multiple muscle groups simultaneously, making them a valuable addition to any strength-training routine. In this section, we will explore the proper technique and benefits of push-ups.

How to Perform Push-Ups:

1. Start by positioning yourself face down on the floor, with your hands slightly wider than shoulder-width apart. Your toes should be touching the ground, and your body should form a straight line from head to heels.

2. Engage your core by drawing your navel in toward your spine. This will help maintain a stable and aligned body position throughout the exercise.

3. Lower your body toward the floor by bending your elbows, keeping them close to your sides. Lower yourself until your chest nearly touches the ground, or as far as you can comfortably go without straining.

4. Pause briefly at the bottom of the movement, then exhale and push through your hands to extend your arms

and return to the starting position. Keep your body straight and avoid sagging or arching your back.

5. Repeat the movement for the desired number of repetitions, typically 8 to 12, depending on your fitness level and goals.

Tips for Performing Push-Ups:

- Maintain a neutral spine throughout the exercise by keeping your head in line with your body. Avoid looking up or tucking your chin.
- Keep your core muscles engaged throughout the movement to provide stability and prevent your lower back from sagging.
- Focus on a controlled and smooth motion, avoiding jerky or fast movements.
- Modify the exercise if needed by performing push-ups on your knees or against an elevated surface, such as a bench or wall, until you build enough strength to perform full push-ups.
- Gradually increase the difficulty by progressing to more challenging variations, such as diamond push-ups, decline push-ups, or one-arm push-ups.

Benefits of Push-Ups:

- Upper Body Strength: Push-ups target the muscles of the chest, shoulders, and triceps, helping to build strength and definition in these areas.
- Core Activation: Push-ups engage the core muscles, including the abdominals and lower back, to stabilize the body throughout the exercise.
- Functional Fitness: Push-ups simulate movements used in various activities, such as pushing objects or performing activities that require upper body strength, making them highly functional.
- Convenience and Versatility: Push-ups can be performed anywhere, requiring no equipment. They can be easily modified to accommodate different fitness levels and goals.
- Improved Posture: Regularly performing push-ups can help improve posture by strengthening the muscles of the upper back and shoulders, which are essential for maintaining proper alignment.

Pull-Ups

Pull-ups are a challenging and effective strength-training exercise that primarily targets the muscles of the upper body, particularly the back, shoulders, and arms. They are a compound exercise that requires the use of multiple muscle groups, making them a valuable addition to any strength-training routine. In this section, we will explore the proper technique and benefits of pull-ups.

How to Perform Pull-Ups:

1. Find a sturdy overhead bar or pull-up bar that can support your body weight. Grasp the bar with an overhand grip, slightly wider than shoulder-width apart.

2. Hang from the bar with your arms fully extended, and your body relaxed.

3. Engage your core muscles and squeeze your shoulder blades together. This will help stabilize your body throughout the movement.

4. Pull yourself up by bending your arms, leading with your elbows. Focus on using your back muscles to initiate the movement.

5. Continue pulling until your chin is above the level of the bar. Maintain control and avoid swinging or using momentum.

6. Slowly lower yourself back down to the starting position, fully extending your arms.

7. Repeat the movement for the desired number of repetitions, typically 5 to 10, depending on your fitness level and goals.

Tips for Performing Pull-Ups:

- Start with a grip that feels comfortable and allows you to maintain proper form. You can experiment with different grip variations, such as overhand (pronated), underhand (supinated), or mixed grip.
- Keep your body straight and avoid swinging or using your legs to assist with the movement. Focus on using your upper body muscles to pull yourself up.
- Control the descent and avoid dropping down quickly. Maintain tension in your muscles throughout the entire range of motion.
- If you are unable to perform a full pull-up, you can start with assisted pull-ups using a resistance band or an assisted pull-up machine. Alternatively, you can perform negative pull-ups by focusing on the lowering phase of the movement.

- Gradually increase the difficulty by progressing to more challenging variations, such as wide-grip pull-ups, close-grip pull-ups, or weighted pull-ups.

Benefits of Pull-Ups:

- *Upper Body Strength:* Pull-ups target the muscles of the upper body, including the back, shoulders, and arms, helping to develop strength and muscular endurance in these areas.
- *Back Development:* Pull-ups specifically target the muscles of the back, including the latissimus dorsi, rhomboids, and trapezius, promoting a strong and defined back.
- *Core Activation:* Pull-ups require core engagement to stabilise the body during the movement, contributing to improved core strength and stability.
- *Grip Strength:* Pull-ups challenge the grip strength, which is beneficial for various activities and sports that require grip endurance and control.
- *Functional Movement:* Pull-ups simulate pulling movements used in daily life, such as lifting objects or pulling oneself up over obstacles, making them highly functional.

Chapter 7

Balance Exercises

Standing on One Leg

Balance exercises are an essential component of any well-rounded fitness routine, particularly for individuals with osteoporosis. These exercises help improve stability, coordination, and proprioception, which is the body's sense of its position in space. In this section, we will explore one of the fundamental balance exercises: standing on one leg.

How to Perform Standing on One Leg:

1. Stand tall with your feet hip-width apart, arms relaxed at your sides, and your gaze fixed on a focal point in front of you.

2. Shift your weight onto one leg while maintaining a soft bend in the knee. The other foot should be lifted slightly off the ground, with the toes pointed forward.

3. Engage your core muscles and find your balance by focusing on your body's alignment and stability.

4. Hold this position for a specific duration, typically starting with 10 to 30 seconds, or as long as you can maintain good form and balance.

5. Switch to the other leg and repeat the exercise for the same duration.

Tips for Performing Standing on One Leg:

- Keep your standing leg slightly bent to maintain stability and prevent locking the knee.
- If you find it challenging to balance initially, you can lightly touch a wall, chair, or countertop for support until you gain more confidence and stability.
- Focus on a fixed point in front of you to help improve your balance and prevent dizziness or disorientation.
- Engage your core muscles by drawing your navel towards your spine, which will help improve your overall stability and balance.
- Breathe deeply and maintain a relaxed posture throughout the exercise.

Benefits of Standing on One Leg:

- Improved Balance and Stability: Standing on one leg challenges your balance and trains your body to stabilize itself, which can help prevent falls and enhance overall stability in daily activities.

- Enhanced Proprioception: By performing balance exercises like standing on one leg, you improve your body's ability to sense its position in space, promoting better coordination and body awareness.

- Strengthening Leg Muscles: This exercise targets the muscles of the standing leg, including the quadriceps, hamstrings, calf muscles, and ankle stabilizers, helping to build strength and endurance.

- Core Activation: Maintaining proper balance requires engaging your core muscles, including the abdominals and lower back, which contributes to improved core strength and stability.

- Functional Movement: Enhancing your balance through exercises like standing on one leg can translate into improved performance in activities that require stability, such as walking, climbing stairs, or participating in sports.

Tai Chi

Tai Chi is a traditional Chinese martial art that incorporates flowing movements, deep breathing, and mental focus. It is widely recognized for its numerous health benefits, including improving balance and stability. In this section, we will explore the practice of Tai Chi as a balance exercise and its potential benefits for individuals with osteoporosis.

What is Tai Chi?

Tai Chi originated as a martial art but has evolved into a gentle, low-impact exercise suitable for people of all ages and fitness levels. It consists of a series of slow, continuous movements performed in a mindful and controlled manner. These movements are typically combined with deep breathing and a relaxed state of mind. Tai Chi focuses on cultivating balance, flexibility, strength, and coordination while promoting overall well-being.

How Tai Chi Improves Balance:

1. Weight Shift: Tai Chi incorporates weight shifting from one leg to another, which helps improve proprioception, balance control, and stability.

2. Body Alignment: The postures and movements in Tai Chi promote proper body alignment and posture, enhancing balance and reducing the risk of falls.

3. Lower Body Strength: Tai Chi involves controlled leg movements, deep stances, and shifting weight, which can strengthen the muscles in the lower body, including the legs, hips, and ankles.

4. Core Stability: The slow and deliberate movements in Tai Chi engage the core muscles, including the abdominals and back muscles, which contribute to better balance and stability.

5. Mind-Body Connection: Tai Chi emphasises mindfulness and focus, enabling individuals to develop a heightened sense of body awareness, coordination, and balance.

Benefits of Tai Chi for Balance:

- Improved Balance and Stability: The practice of Tai Chi helps improve balance control, reducing the risk of falls and enhancing stability in daily activities.

- Increased Flexibility: Tai Chi incorporates gentle stretches and flowing movements, which can improve joint flexibility and range of motion, contributing to better balance and mobility.

- *Enhanced Posture and Body Alignment:* Tai Chi promotes proper body alignment and posture, helping to alleviate muscle imbalances and reduce strain on joints, leading to improved balance.

- *Stress Reduction:* Tai Chi combines physical movement with mental relaxation and deep breathing, promoting a sense of calmness and reducing stress levels. This can indirectly contribute to improved balance by reducing muscle tension and promoting a more focused state of mind.

- *Overall Well-being:* Practising Tai Chi has been associated with various health benefits, including improved cardiovascular fitness, increased energy levels, and better mental well-being.

Yoga

Yoga is an ancient practice that combines physical postures, breathing techniques, and meditation to promote physical, mental, and spiritual well-being. In addition to its many benefits for flexibility, strength, and stress reduction, yoga also offers a variety of balance exercises that can help improve stability and coordination. In this section, we will explore the practice of yoga as a balance exercise and its potential benefits for individuals with osteoporosis.

What is Yoga?

Yoga originated in ancient India and has since gained popularity worldwide as a holistic approach to health and wellness. It involves performing a series of poses or asanas, along with controlled breathing and mindfulness. Yoga encompasses various styles, such as Hatha, Vinyasa, and Iyengar, each with its own emphasis and approach.

How Yoga Improves Balance:

1. Body Awareness: Yoga practice cultivates body awareness by encouraging individuals to focus on their alignment, balance, and sensations within each pose.

This heightened awareness helps improve balance control and proprioception.

2. Core Strength: Many yoga poses engage the core muscles, including the abdominals and back muscles, which are essential for maintaining balance and stability.

3. Leg Strength: Yoga poses often require standing on one leg or maintaining stable positions, which helps strengthen the leg muscles, including the quadriceps, hamstrings, and calves.

4. Stability and Flexibility: Yoga poses challenge both stability and flexibility, requiring individuals to find a balance between strength and ease. Through consistent practice, this can lead to improved overall balance and range of motion.

5. Mind-Body Connection: Yoga emphasizes the integration of breath, movement, and mindfulness. By cultivating a focused and present state of mind, individuals develop a stronger mind-body connection, enhancing balance and coordination.

Benefits of Yoga for Balance:

- *Improved Balance and Stability:* Regular yoga practice helps improve balance, coordination, and stability, reducing the risk of falls and enhancing overall body control.

- *Increased Flexibility:* Yoga incorporates gentle stretching and lengthening of muscles, promoting flexibility, which is crucial for maintaining balance and preventing injuries.

- *Core Strength and Stability:* Yoga poses activate and strengthen the core muscles, providing a stable foundation for balance and improving overall posture.

- *Stress Reduction:* The combination of physical movement, controlled breathing, and mindfulness in yoga promotes relaxation and stress reduction. Lower stress levels can indirectly contribute to better balance by reducing muscle tension and promoting mental clarity.

- *Body Alignment and Posture:* Yoga encourages proper body alignment, leading to improved posture and reduced strain on joints. This alignment contributes to better balance and stability.

Walking on a Balance Beam

Walking on a balance beam is a simple yet effective balance exercise that can help improve stability, coordination, and proprioception. While it may seem like a basic activity, walking on a narrow surface challenges your balance control and engages the muscles involved in maintaining stability. In this section, we will explore the benefits of walking on a balance beam as a balance exercise and how it can be incorporated into your routine.

What is a Balance Beam?

A balance beam is a long, narrow platform that is raised off the ground, typically made of wood or other sturdy materials. It is commonly used in gymnastics and other athletic training to enhance balance, body control, and spatial awareness. In the context of balance exercises for osteoporosis, a balance beam can be a modified version suitable for home use.

How Walking on a Balance Beam Improves Balance:

1. Balance and Stability: Walking on a narrow surface like a balance beam challenges your balance and requires you to engage your core muscles and lower body to maintain stability.

2. Proprioception: Walking on a balance beam enhances your proprioception, which is your body's awareness of its position in space. This increased awareness helps improve balance control and coordination.

3. Leg Strength: The act of walking on a balance beam engages the muscles in your legs, including the calves, quadriceps, and hamstrings, helping to strengthen them over time.

4. Concentration and Focus: Walking on a narrow surface requires concentration and focus, as you need to pay attention to your body's movements and maintain a steady stride. This can enhance your mental focus and concentration skills.

Benefits of Walking on a Balance Beam for Balance:

- Improved Balance and Coordination: Walking on a balance beam challenges your balance and coordination, helping to improve your overall stability and reducing the risk of falls.

- Core Strength: Walking on a narrow surface engages your core muscles, including the abdominals and back muscles, promoting core strength and stability.

- Leg Strength and Endurance: The act of walking on a balance beam activates and strengthens the muscles in your legs, enhancing their strength and endurance.

- Enhanced Proprioception: Walking on a narrow surface like a balance beam enhances your body's proprioceptive abilities, improving your sense of balance and spatial awareness.

- Functional Balance: Walking on a balance beam can translate to improved balance and stability in your everyday activities, such as walking on uneven surfaces or navigating stairs.

Incorporating walking on a balance beam into your balance exercise routine can be a fun and effective way to enhance your balance, stability, and coordination. You can start by using a low and stable beam, gradually progressing to narrower and more challenging surfaces as your skills improve. Ensure that the beam is secure and safe to use, and consider having a spotter or using handrails for added support. It's important to start with shorter durations and gradually increase the time spent on the beam as your confidence and balance improve.

Chapter 8

Putting It All Together

Creating a Personalized Exercise Plan

Now that you have explored various weight-bearing, strength-training, and balance exercises, it's time to bring everything together and create a personalised exercise plan that suits your needs and goals. Having a well-designed plan will help you stay consistent, track your progress, and maximise the benefits of your workouts. In this section, we will guide you through the process of creating your personalised exercise plan for osteoporosis management.

Assessing Your Goals:

Before creating your exercise plan, it's essential to assess your goals. What do you want to achieve through your exercise routine? Are you primarily focused on improving bone density, reducing the risk of fractures, increasing strength and stability, or enhancing overall fitness and well-being? Understanding your goals will help you choose the most appropriate exercises and set realistic expectations.

Next, consider your current health condition and fitness level. Take into account any specific recommendations or restrictions provided by your healthcare provider. If you have any underlying medical conditions or limitations, it's crucial to tailor your exercise plan accordingly and consult with your healthcare professional if needed.

Exercise Components:

Your exercise plan should include a combination of weight-bearing exercises, strength-training exercises, and balance exercises. Select exercises from the respective chapters that align with your goals and preferences. Aim for a well-rounded routine that targets different muscle groups and aspects of bone health and balance.

Frequency and Duration:

Determine how often you will engage in exercise and the duration of each session. It's generally recommended to engage in weight-bearing exercises at least 3-4 times per week, strength-training exercises 2-3 times per week, and balance exercises 2-3 times per week. Start with a duration that feels comfortable for you and gradually increase it as you build strength and endurance.

Progression and Modification:

As you become more comfortable with your exercise routine, you can gradually increase the intensity, duration, or difficulty of certain exercises. This progressive approach helps to challenge your body and promote further improvements. Additionally, be open to modifications or alternative exercises based on your individual needs, preferences, and any physical limitations you may have.

Safety Measures:

Ensure that your exercise plan incorporates safety measures to reduce the risk of injuries. This includes proper warm-up and cool-down routines, using appropriate footwear and equipment, maintaining proper form and technique, and listening to your body's signals. If you experience pain or discomfort during an exercise, modify or stop the movement and seek guidance if necessary.

Tracking Your Progress:

Lastly, consider how you will track your progress. This can be done through various methods such as keeping an exercise journal, using fitness apps, or utilizing wearable fitness trackers. Regularly assess your progress, celebrate milestones, and make adjustments to your exercise plan as needed.

Remember, it's important to listen to your body, start gradually, and seek guidance from qualified professionals, such as exercise physiologists or physical therapists, if necessary. They can provide additional expertise and ensure that your exercise plan is safe and effective.

By creating a personalized exercise plan, you are taking a proactive step towards managing osteoporosis and improving your bone health. Stay committed, stay consistent, and enjoy the benefits that regular exercise can bring to your overall well-being.

Incorporating Different Exercises

In order to maximise the benefits of your exercise routine and keep it engaging and enjoyable, it's important to incorporate a variety of different exercises. By including exercises from different categories, such as weight-bearing, strength-training, and balance exercises, you can target different aspects of bone health, muscle strength, and overall fitness. In this section, we will explore the importance of incorporating different exercises and provide practical tips for diversifying your workouts.

Benefits of Variety in Exercise:

1. Comprehensive Bone Health: Different exercises put varying degrees of stress on your bones, helping to stimulate bone remodeling and improve bone density. By incorporating a mix of weight-bearing and strength-training exercises, you can provide a comprehensive approach to bone health.

2. Muscular Strength and Endurance: Different exercises engage different muscle groups, allowing you to target and strengthen various areas of your body. This promotes overall muscular strength, endurance, and functional fitness.

3. Balance and Coordination: Balance exercises challenge your stability and proprioception, enhancing your balance and reducing the risk of falls. By including balance exercises in your routine, you can improve your coordination and stability.

4. Psychological Benefits: Engaging in a variety of exercises prevents monotony and boredom, making your workouts more enjoyable. This can lead to increased motivation, adherence, and overall psychological well-being.

Tips for Incorporating Different Exercises:

1. Rotate Exercise Categories: Plan your workouts to include a mix of weight-bearing exercises, strength-training exercises, and balance exercises. For example, you could dedicate certain days of the week to each category or alternate between them throughout the week.

2. Vary Intensity and Difficulty: Within each exercise category, vary the intensity and difficulty levels. For weight-bearing exercises, you can choose between low-impact and high-impact options. With strength-training exercises, progress from lighter weights to heavier weights or try different variations of the exercises to challenge your muscles in new ways. For balance exercises, you can start with basic movements and gradually advance to more complex ones.

3. *Explore Different Modalities:* Within each exercise category, explore different modalities or variations. For example, if you enjoy walking as a weight-bearing exercise, you can mix it up by trying different terrains, walking at different speeds, or using a treadmill or elliptical machine. Similarly, if you enjoy strength-training exercises, experiment with different types of resistance, such as free weights, resistance bands, or weight machines.

4. *Incorporate Group Classes or Workouts:* Consider joining group classes or workout sessions that offer a variety of exercises. This can include fitness classes, dance classes, yoga sessions, or sports activities. Group settings provide an opportunity to learn new exercises, engage with others, and add a social element to your exercise routine.

5. *Listen to Your Body:* Pay attention to how your body responds to different exercises. Some exercises may feel more comfortable and enjoyable, while others may cause discomfort or strain. Adjust your exercise choices accordingly and consult with a healthcare professional or fitness instructor if you have any concerns.

Progression and Modification

As you continue with your exercise plan for osteoporosis management, it's important to incorporate progression and modification to challenge your body, prevent plateauing, and ensure continued improvements. Progression involves gradually increasing the intensity, duration, or difficulty of your exercises, while modification allows you to adapt exercises based on your individual needs and capabilities. In this section, we will explore the concepts of progression and modification and provide guidance on how to effectively implement them in your exercise routine.

The Importance of Progression:

Progression is crucial for optimising the benefits of your exercises. By gradually increasing the demands on your body, you can stimulate further improvements in bone density, muscle strength, balance, and overall fitness. Progression also helps to keep your workouts challenging and interesting, preventing boredom and maintaining motivation.

Tips for Progression:

1. Increase Intensity: Gradually increase the intensity of your exercises. For weight-bearing exercises, this can involve walking at a faster pace, jogging instead of walking, or incorporating hills or inclines. For strength-training exercises, increase the resistance by using heavier weights, resistance bands with higher tension, or performing more repetitions or sets.

2. Extend Duration: Gradually extend the duration of your workouts. For weight-bearing exercises, aim to walk or engage in other weight-bearing activities for longer periods of time. For strength-training exercises, increase the number of sets or repetitions you perform. Balancing exercises can also be extended by holding poses for longer durations.

3. Add Variation: Introduce new exercises or variations of existing exercises to challenge your body in different ways. For example, you can try different types of lunges, squats, or yoga poses. Adding variation keeps your muscles guessing and promotes well-rounded fitness.

4. Incorporate Interval Training: Interval training involves alternating between periods of higher intensity and lower intensity or rest. This can be applied to both cardiovascular exercises, such as jogging or cycling, and strength-training exercises. Interval training boosts cardiovascular fitness, burns more calories, and provides a new level of challenge.

Modification allows you to adapt exercises to suit your individual needs, limitations, and abilities. It ensures that you can safely engage in exercises while still benefiting from them. Modification is particularly important if you have specific health concerns, physical limitations, or are recovering from an injury.

Tips for Modification:

1. Focus on Proper Form: Always prioritise maintaining proper form and technique during exercises. This helps to prevent injuries and ensures that you are targeting the intended muscles effectively. If you're unsure about proper form, consider seeking guidance from a qualified fitness professional.

2. Use Supportive Equipment: Utilise supportive equipment, such as exercise bands, stability balls, or balance aids, to assist you in performing exercises with proper form and stability. These tools can provide assistance, stability, or added resistance as needed.

*3. **Adjust Range of Motion:*** Modify exercises by adjusting the range of motion to accommodate your comfort level and joint mobility. You can gradually increase the range of motion as your flexibility and strength improve.

*4. **Seek Professional Guidance:*** If you have specific health concerns or physical limitations, it's beneficial to consult with a healthcare professional, such as a physical therapist or exercise physiologist. They can provide tailored modifications and guidance based on your individual needs.

Remember, both progression and modification are individualised processes. Progress at a pace that feels challenging but manageable for you. Listen to your body and make adjustments as needed. By incorporating progression and modification into your exercise routine, you can ensure continuous improvements while prioritising safety and your unique circumstances.

Staying Motivated

Maintaining motivation is key to sustaining an exercise routine for osteoporosis management. As with any long-term commitment, there may be times when your motivation wanes or obstacles arise. However, by implementing strategies to stay motivated, you can overcome challenges and continue on the path to improved bone health and overall well-being. In this section, we will explore various techniques to help you stay motivated and committed to your exercise plan.

1. Set Realistic and Achievable Goals: Establish specific, realistic, and achievable goals for your exercise routine. Break down your larger goals into smaller, manageable milestones. Celebrate your accomplishments along the way, which will provide a sense of achievement and motivate you to continue.

2. Find an Exercise Buddy or Support System: Partnering with a friend, family member, or support group can greatly enhance motivation. Having someone to exercise with provides accountability, encouragement, and the opportunity to enjoy physical activity together.

3. Vary Your Routine: Keep your exercise routine interesting and enjoyable by incorporating a variety of exercises. Try new activities, explore different workout locations, or participate in group classes to add excitement and prevent boredom.

4. Track Your Progress: Keep a record of your workouts, including the exercises performed, duration, and any improvements you notice. Tracking your progress can help you visualise your achievements and serve as a reminder of how far you've come.

5. Reward Yourself: Establish a system of rewards for reaching milestones or sticking to your exercise routine. Treat yourself to something you enjoy, such as a relaxing massage, a new workout outfit, or a day off from your usual responsibilities.

6. Find Activities You Enjoy: Engage in exercises that you genuinely enjoy. If you find joy in the activities you participate in, you're more likely to stay motivated and committed. Experiment with different exercises until you discover the ones that bring you pleasure and satisfaction.

7. Create a Supportive Environment: Make your environment conducive to exercise by removing barriers and creating a dedicated space for physical activity. Surround yourself with motivational cues, such as inspirational quotes or images, to remind you of your goals.

8. Use Technology and Apps: Utilise fitness apps, activity trackers, or online communities to stay connected, monitor your progress, and access additional resources. These technological tools can provide motivation, track your achievements, and offer support.

9. Embrace Mind-Body Connection: Incorporate mindfulness techniques, such as meditation or deep breathing exercises, into your exercise routine. Cultivating a mind-body connection can enhance your overall experience and help you stay present and focused.

10. Seek Professional Guidance: Consult with a qualified exercise professional, such as a certified personal trainer or exercise physiologist, to receive expert guidance, individualised exercise plans, and ongoing support. Their expertise can help you stay motivated and ensure that you are safely progressing toward your goals.

Remember, motivation may fluctuate over time, but by implementing these strategies, you can maintain a consistent exercise routine for long-term success. Celebrate your achievements, enjoy the process, and stay focused on the positive impact that regular exercise can have on your bone health and overall quality of life.

Chapter 9

Monitoring Your Progress

Tracking Your Exercise Routine

Monitoring your progress is an essential component of your osteoporosis exercise plan. By tracking your exercise routine, you can gain valuable insights into your performance, stay accountable to your goals, and make necessary adjustments for continued improvement. In this section, we will explore the importance of tracking your exercise routine and provide practical tips for effective monitoring.

Why Track Your Exercise Routine?

Tracking your exercise routine offers several benefits:

1. Accountability: When you record your workouts, you create a sense of accountability. Knowing that you are keeping track of your progress can motivate you to stay consistent and committed to your exercise routine.

2. *Progress Evaluation:* Tracking allows you to evaluate your progress over time. By comparing your current performance to previous data, you can objectively assess improvements in your strength, endurance, balance, or flexibility.

3. *Identifying Patterns:* Monitoring your exercise routine helps you identify patterns or trends. You can observe which exercises or activities yield the most positive results for your bone health and overall fitness. This knowledge allows you to make informed decisions and focus on areas that require attention.

4. *Goal Setting:* Tracking provides a clear picture of your achievements, enabling you to set realistic and attainable goals. By reviewing your progress, you can establish new targets that align with your desired outcomes.

Tips for Effective Tracking:

1. *Choose a Recording Method:* Determine a recording method that works best for you. You can use a paper journal, a spreadsheet, a mobile app, or an online platform designed for exercise tracking. Select a format that is convenient and easily accessible for regular updates.

2. Record Essential Details: Note down essential details for each workout, including the date, duration, exercises performed, sets, repetitions, weights used (if applicable), and any additional notes or observations. The more specific and detailed your recording, the better you can evaluate your progress.

3. Consider Measurements and Assessments: Periodically include measurements and assessments to track changes in your body composition, bone density, or physical capabilities. These may include weight, body measurements, balance assessments, or bone density scans conducted by healthcare professionals.

4. Set Regular Checkpoints: Establish regular checkpoints to review your progress. This can be weekly, biweekly, or monthly, depending on your preference. During these checkpoints, analyse your recorded data, assess your achievements, and set new goals for the upcoming period.

5. Celebrate Milestones: Celebrate milestones along your journey. Acknowledge and reward yourself for reaching specific milestones or achieving significant improvements. This positive reinforcement can boost motivation and foster a sense of accomplishment.

6. *Reflect on Challenges and Adjustments:* Use your tracking records to reflect on any challenges or obstacles you encountered during your exercise routine. Assess what worked well and what areas need improvement. Make adjustments to your plan accordingly, such as modifying exercises, increasing intensity, or seeking professional guidance.

7. *Share Your Progress:* Consider sharing your progress with a trusted friend, family member, or support group. Sharing your achievements and challenges can provide encouragement, support, and additional accountability.

Assessing Improvements in Bone Health

As you engage in weight-bearing exercises to strengthen your bones and reduce the risk of fractures, it is essential to assess your progress in terms of bone health. Monitoring and assessing improvements in your bone health can provide valuable feedback on the effectiveness of your exercise routine and guide further interventions. In this section, we will explore methods for assessing improvements in bone health and understanding the significance of these assessments.

Methods for Assessing Bone Health:

1. Bone Density Scans: Bone density scans, such as dual-energy X-ray absorptiometry (DXA), are commonly used to measure bone mineral density (BMD). These scans provide a numerical value that indicates the density of your bones, which can help evaluate your risk of fractures and monitor changes over time.

2. Fracture Risk Assessment: Your healthcare provider can conduct a fracture risk assessment using tools like the FRAX® algorithm. This assessment takes into account multiple factors, including age, sex, weight, height, previous fractures, and BMD results, to estimate your probability of experiencing a fracture in the next 10 years.

3. Biochemical Markers: Certain blood or urine tests can measure biochemical markers related to bone turnover. These markers indicate the rate at which bone formation and resorption occur in your body. Changes in these markers can provide insights into your bone metabolism and response to exercise.

4. Functional Assessments: Functional assessments evaluate your physical abilities and functional performance, which indirectly reflect improvements in bone health. These assessments may include measures of strength, balance, flexibility, mobility, and posture.

Interpreting the Assessments:

Interpreting the assessments requires collaboration with your healthcare provider or an expert in bone health. They will help you understand the results and their implications for your bone health. Here are some key considerations:

1. Baseline Measurements: Establishing baseline measurements allows for comparison over time. The initial assessments provide a starting point for evaluating improvements and identifying areas that require further attention.

2. *Longitudinal Analysis:* Comparing assessments conducted at different time points helps determine if your exercise routine is positively impacting your bone health. Longitudinal analysis allows you to observe trends, assess the rate of change, and make necessary adjustments to your exercise plan.

3. *Individual Variability:* It's important to note that individual responses to exercise can vary. Some individuals may experience more significant improvements in bone health, while others may show a slower rate of change. Your healthcare provider will consider your unique circumstances and provide personalised guidance based on your assessments.

4. *Additional Factors:* Assessments provide valuable insights, but it's crucial to consider other factors that contribute to overall bone health, such as nutrition, hormonal balance, medication use, and lifestyle choices. Evaluating these factors alongside your assessments will offer a comprehensive view of your bone health.

Seeking Professional Guidance

When engaging in weight-bearing exercises for osteoporosis and monitoring your progress, seeking professional guidance is crucial for accurate assessments and personalised recommendations. Healthcare professionals, such as doctors, physiotherapists, or exercise specialists, can provide expert insight and support throughout your journey. In this section, we will discuss the importance of seeking professional guidance and how they can assist you in monitoring your progress effectively.

The Importance of Professional Guidance:

1. Expertise in Osteoporosis Management: Healthcare professionals specialised in osteoporosis have in-depth knowledge and expertise in managing the condition. They can help you understand the unique challenges associated with osteoporosis, tailor exercises to your specific needs, and guide you on the most effective and safe ways to strengthen your bones.

2. Personalised Assessment: Professionals can conduct comprehensive assessments to evaluate your bone health, functional abilities, and overall fitness. They may use tools such as bone density scans, functional tests, and medical history analysis to gain a complete understanding of your condition and track your progress accurately.

3. Individualised Exercise Recommendations: Based on your assessments, healthcare professionals can provide personalised exercise recommendations that consider your current fitness level, bone health status, and any specific limitations or contraindications you may have. They can guide you in selecting appropriate exercises, modifying movements, and gradually progressing your exercise routine.

4. Safety and Injury Prevention: Professionals can ensure that you perform exercises with proper form and technique, reducing the risk of injuries. They can educate you about safety considerations, teach you how to use exercise equipment correctly, and provide guidance on proper warm-up and cool-down routines.

5. Monitoring and Adjustment: Healthcare professionals can monitor your progress over time, analyse the results of your assessments, and make necessary adjustments to your exercise plan. They can identify areas that need improvement, offer guidance on exercise progression, and help you set realistic goals for optimal bone health.

6. Holistic Approach: Professionals can take a holistic approach to your bone health, considering other factors such as nutrition, medication management, and lifestyle modifications. They can provide recommendations on dietary changes, supplementation, and lifestyle habits that support your exercise routine and overall well-being.

How to Seek Professional Guidance:

1. Consult with your Doctor: Start by consulting with your primary care physician or an osteoporosis specialist. They can refer you to the appropriate healthcare professionals, such as physiotherapists or exercise specialists, who have experience in managing osteoporosis.

2. Choose Qualified Professionals: Look for professionals who have experience and expertise in osteoporosis management and exercise prescription. They should be knowledgeable about the latest research and guidelines related to osteoporosis and have a track record of working with individuals with similar needs.

3. Open Communication: Maintain open and honest communication with your healthcare professionals. Share any concerns, limitations, or changes in your health status that may affect your exercise routine. This will ensure that they have all the necessary information to provide you with the best guidance and support.

4. *Regular Follow-ups:* Schedule regular follow-up appointments with your healthcare professionals to track your progress, review assessments, and receive ongoing guidance. These appointments are an opportunity to discuss any challenges, ask questions, and receive further recommendations for optimising your bone health.

Conclusion

Weight-bearing exercises offer numerous benefits for individuals with osteoporosis, including strengthening bones and reducing the risk of fractures. Throughout this book, we have explored the scientific evidence supporting the effectiveness of weight-bearing exercises in managing osteoporosis and improving bone health. By incorporating these exercises into your daily routine, you can take proactive steps towards enhancing your bone strength and overall well-being.

Weight-bearing exercises work by applying stress to your bones, stimulating the process of bone remodeling. This process leads to increased bone density and improved bone quality, making your bones stronger and more resilient. Additionally, these exercises enhance muscle strength, improve balance and coordination, and promote overall fitness. They not only contribute to better bone health but also support your overall physical function and independence.

In this book, we have covered a variety of low-impact and high-impact weight-bearing exercises, including walking, dancing, water aerobics, Tai Chi, yoga, jogging, jumping rope, tennis, basketball, and hiking. We have also explored strength-training exercises and balance exercises that complement the weight-bearing exercises for a well-rounded exercise routine.

To ensure your safety and maximise the benefits of these exercises, it is important to consult with your healthcare provider and seek professional guidance. Qualified exercise instructors or physiotherapists with expertise in osteoporosis management can help you develop a personalised exercise plan, assess your fitness level, provide proper guidance on exercise techniques, and monitor your progress. Their knowledge and support will help you navigate the journey towards stronger bones effectively and minimise the risk of injury.

Remember, consistency is key when it comes to reaping the benefits of weight-bearing exercises. By incorporating these exercises into your daily routine and gradually progressing your intensity and duration, you can make significant strides in improving your bone health and reducing the risk of fractures. Stay motivated, listen to your body, and make adjustments as needed to ensure that your exercise routine remains enjoyable and sustainable.

In conclusion, weight-bearing exercises are a scientifically proven approach to strengthen your bones and reduce the risk of fractures associated with osteoporosis. By implementing the exercises outlined in this book, seeking professional guidance, and staying committed to your exercise routine, you are taking proactive steps towards better bone health and a higher quality of life. Embrace the journey, enjoy the benefits, and empower yourself to live an active and fulfilling life with strong and resilient bones.

Finding a qualified exercise instructor or physiotherapist can be instrumental in your osteoporosis exercise journey. Consider the following steps to find the right professional for your needs:

1. Seek Recommendations: Ask your healthcare provider, friends, or support groups for recommendations on qualified exercise instructors who specialise in osteoporosis management. They may have valuable insights based on personal experiences or professional connections.

2. Research Credentials and Experience: Look for professionals who have relevant certifications, such as certifications in exercise science, physiotherapy, or osteoporosis management. Check their experience and inquire about their familiarity with working with individuals with osteoporosis.

3. Assess Knowledge of Osteoporosis: During your initial consultation or interview, assess the instructor's knowledge and understanding of osteoporosis. They should be familiar with the condition, its impact on bone health, and the specific exercise considerations and modifications required for individuals with osteoporosis.

4. Communication and Rapport: Effective communication and a positive rapport with your exercise instructor are essential for a successful working relationship. Ensure that they listen to your concerns, understand your goals, and are responsive to your questions and feedback.

5. Personalised Approach: Look for an instructor who emphasises a personalised approach to exercise programming. They should consider your unique needs, abilities, and limitations, and tailor the exercise program accordingly. This individualised approach will help maximise the benefits and minimise the risk of injury.

Remember, finding a qualified exercise instructor is an investment in your bone health and overall well-being. By working with a professional who understands the intricacies of osteoporosis and exercise, you can feel confident in the guidance and support you receive throughout your journey.

In closing, this book has provided you with valuable insights into the benefits of weight-bearing exercises for osteoporosis, the importance of seeking professional guidance, and practical guidelines for incorporating these exercises into your routine. Armed with this knowledge, you can embark on your journey towards stronger bones, reduced fracture risk, and a more active and fulfilling life. Embrace the power of weight-bearing exercises, take control of your bone health, and enjoy the lifelong benefits they offer.

Made in the USA
Las Vegas, NV
13 March 2024

87119494R10075